The Ultimate
Keto Chaffle Recipes
Cookbook

Quick And Easy Recipes To Burn Fat And Boost Your Brain Health.

Diana Humble

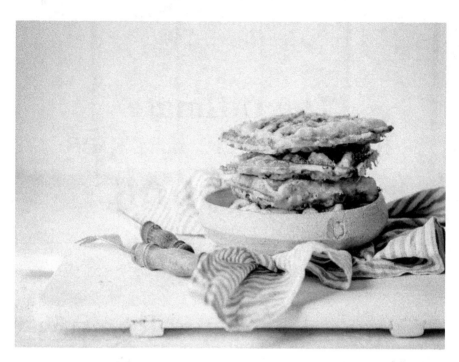

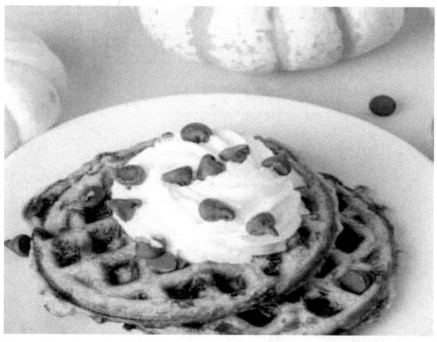

TABLE OF CONTENTS

allowed with the express written consent from the Publisher. All additional right reserved.

The information in the following pages is broadly considered a truthful and accurate account of facts and as such, any inattention, use, or misuse of the information in question by the reader will render any resulting actions solely under their purview. There are no scenarios in which the publisher or the original author of this work can be in any fashion deemed liable for any hardship or damages that may befall them after undertaking information described herein.

Additionally, the information in the following pages is intended only for informational purposes and should thus be thought of as universal. As befitting its nature, it is presented without assurance regarding its prolonged validity or interim quality. Trademarks that are mentioned are done without written consent and can in no way be considered an endorsement from the trademark holder.

INTRODUCTION

Keto Diet is a high-fat, low-carb diet that is an increasingly popular way to lose weight. Keto is short for "ketosis", which occurs when the body has depleted its sugar stores, so it burns stored fat instead of glucose in order to produce energy.

Losing weight on a keto diet sounds pretty easy; just eat a few bacon sandwiches and you'll be slimmer in no time. However, there are drawbacks to this diet, including very low levels of vegetables and fruit (so important for fiber and other nutrients) as well as constipation from lack of dietary fiber. Here are some tips:

- It's important to drink plenty of water, not only because you may be eating more sodium than you need, but because staying hydrated will help your body process proteins and fats more efficiently.

- For best results, stay away from most fruits and vegetables. Some berries are allowed; others aren't. Vegetables that are considered "low in carbs" or "leafy greens" are fine—but there is a difference between low-carb and high-fiber. As a rule of thumb, if it looks like it has the texture of tree bark or is covered with seeds or bulbs (e.g., artichokes), it probably has a lot of carbs and should be avoided.

- Be careful with spices, which tend to have a lot of sugar; salt is OK. It can be easy to go overboard on spices.

- Eat plenty of salmon, tuna and egg whites. Meat—including beef, chicken, pork and lamb—should comprise 20 to 25 percent of your total diet. (Be aware that "lean" meat is often not very lean. Be prepared to trim off most of that fat before cooking.) A little bacon or sausage is fine, too.

- Avoid condiments and sauces, including barbecue sauce and ketchup. These are full of sugar and other unhealthy ingredients.

- Drink mostly water (or unsweetened drinks such as tea or coffee). Try to avoid drinks with a lot of added sugar, like fruit juice or alcohol. If you choose to drink wine, go for the dry stuff—red wine is best.

Now, for Chaffles.

What is Chaffle?

Keto chaffle recipe is a versatile and easy-to-make low carb pancake that only requires 2 ingredients. It's a way to satisfy your sweet cravings while staying keto!

Chaffle is made from cheese and eggs. You will need grated cheddar cheese (use any kind of cheese you have on hand) and eggs, beaten together, then fried in a pan with butter or coconut oil.

Chaffles are perfect for a low carb breakfast, lunch or dinner and can be a treat right out of the pan, with butter!

Why Keto and Chaffle is a perfect combination?

Keto Chaffle is a great way to satisfy your sweet cravings while staying 100% in ketosis. It helps you feel fuller for longer but at the same time it's not a high carb treat.

Chaffle gives you a lot of energy and it's an easy way to prepare breakfast if you want it to be ready quickly when you get up or even if you're in a hurry so it can be prepared on the go without any issues.

Keto Chaffle tastes amazing plain, with butter or with any toppings you like and it can also be used as sandwich bread substitute.

KETOGENIC DIET AND ITS BENEFITS

What is Ketogenic Diet?

The ketogenic diet is a low-carb, high-fat diet. This means that the macronutrient ratio of your diet should consist mainly of fat and protein with only a small percentage of carbohydrates.

The idea behind the ketogenic diet is to force your body to use fat rather than glucose as its primary fuel source. When we are in ketosis, we can function on almost any fuel source.

Benefits of the Ketogenic Diet

The benefits of the ketogenic diet are as follows:

1. No need to count calories.

On this diet, you can eat as much as you want. Since there are no grains, the carbohydrates in the diet are very low, and so you will not take in many calories.

2. There is no need to spend a lot of money on expensive foods.

Since this diet is high in fat, one of the cheapest sources of fat is chicken thighs and legs and other skinless poultry parts or meats from around the animal, such as organ meats (heart, liver, etc.).

3. Low levels of Beta-hydroxybutyrate (ketone body) is suitable for brain health

The ketogenic diet can increase the level of ketone bodies by 10 times than normal dietary levels through fat metabolism.

4. Decreased risk of heart disease

Many people can lower their LDL (bad) cholesterol by 75-90% and triglyceride levels by 60%.

5. Less inflammation

Because there are no carbohydrates in the ketogenic diet, your body becomes very efficient at burning ketones as fuel. This is excellent news if you have an autoimmune disorder like rheumatoid arthritis or Crohn's disease because inflammation is often linked to autoimmune problems.

6. Fast weight loss

People usually start losing weight within two weeks of starting the diet.

7. Increased energy levels

The ketogenic diet can increase your energy levels because you will be consuming a high-fat diet with very few carbohydrates.

8. No constant hunger

When people are on a ketogenic diet, they are in "ketosis." This means that their bodies are using fat as an almost complete fuel source. This is the opposite of how most people function in a non-ketogenic state, which usually involves using carbohydrates (sugars) as a practically whole fuel source. Because the ketogenic diet is so different, the body is forced to use fat as its primary fuel source to function. This means you won't be hungry all the time once you get the hang of it.

9. No need for cheat meals

Since carbohydrates are reduced in this diet, cheating on the ketogenic diet will not help you lose weight because your body does not have carbohydrates stored to keep your metabolism running, being that fat is used instead of sugar/carbs.

10. No need to buy expensive supplements

Since the diet is not very restrictive, you won't need to buy many supplements besides vitamin D3 if you are deficient.

11. You can gain muscle and lose fat at the same time

When you do strength training with a ketogenic diet, the weight loss is due to body fat (adipose tissue), not muscle mass. Many people find it difficult to lose weight because they are losing muscle mass and body fat, which is not suitable for overall health. However, because this diet encourages protein consumption at every meal, as well as healthy fats, your amino acid intake will be sufficient to preserve your muscles without inhibiting your weight loss.

Foods Allowed

Here is the list of foods you can eat during the ketogenic diet:

1. Meat, poultry, fish, shellfish, and eggs from pasture-fed animals (animals are fed a grass-fed diet)

2. Fish and seafood caught in the wild

3. Eggs from pastured hens

4. Vegetables, including root vegetables such as beets and carrots and leafy greens such as spinach and kale.

5. Healthy fats such as coconut oil or olive oil that can be used in place of butter or other oils (11 grams per day maximum)

6. Nuts and seeds such as macadamia nuts, walnuts, and pumpkin seeds

7. Low to moderate amounts of dairy products such as yogurt and cheese

8. Non-starchy vegetables such as broccoli, cauliflower, and other cruciferous vegetables

9. Fruits

Foods That Are Not Allowed

Foods that are not allowed

When following the keto diet, you will want to avoid eating the following foods:

1. Grains including wheat, oats, rice, and corn

2. Sugar, including honey, maple syrup, and sugar in all its forms

3. Vegetable oils such as canola, sunflower, and soybean oil

4. Trans fats such as margarine and vegetable shortening

5. Juices and sugary drinks such as soda, fruit juices with added sugar or artificial sweeteners, or milk alternatives made with grains such as almond milk

6. Grain-based dairy products such as butter and yogurt

7. Legumes such as beans, soybeans, and peanuts

8. Starchy vegetables such as potatoes, peas, and corn

9. Processed foods of any kind, including sauces and any food that contains a high percentage of preservatives

10. Beer (pure alcohol)

11. Low-fat or nonfat dairy products such as yogurt and cheese (dairy products that are low in fat but have carbohydrates)

12. Fruit juices with added sugars or artificial sweeteners

Volume (liquid)

US Customary	Metric
1/8 teaspoon	.6 ml
1/4 teaspoon	1.2 ml
1/2 teaspoon	2.5 ml
3/4 teaspoon	3.7 ml
1 teaspoon	5 ml
1 tablespoon	15 ml
2 tablespoon or 1 fluid ounce	30 ml
1/4 cup or 2 fluid ounces	59 ml
1/3 cup	79 ml
1/2 cup	118 ml
2/3 cup	158 ml
3/4 cup	177 ml
1 cup or 8 fluid ounces	237 ml
2 cups or 1 pint	473 ml
4 cups or 1 quart	946 ml
8 cups or 1/2 gallon	1.9 liters
1 gallon	3.8 liters

Weight (mass)

US contemporary (ounces)	Metric (grams)
1/2 ounce	14 grams
1 ounce	28 grams
3 ounces	85 grams
3.53 ounces	100 grams
4 ounces	113 grams
8 ounces	227 grams
12 ounces	340 grams
16 ounces or 1 pound	454 grams

Volume Equivalents (liquid)*

3 teaspoons	1 tablespoon	0.5 fluid ounce
2 tablespoons	1/8 cup	1 fluid ounce
4 tablespoons	1/4 cup	2 fluid ounces
5 1/3 tablespoons	1/3 cup	2.7 fluid ounces
8 tablespoons	1/2 cup	4 fluid ounces
12 tablespoons	3/4 cup	6 fluid ounces
16 tablespoons	1 cup	8 fluid ounces
2 cups	1 pint	16 fluid ounces

BASIC CHAFFLE RECIPES

1. Basic Keto Chaffle Recipe

Preparation Time: 5 minutes

Cooking Time: 8 minutes

Servings: 1

Ingredients:

- 1 egg
- 1/2 cup cheddar cheese, shredded

Directions:

1. Turn waffle maker on or plug it in so that it heats and grease both sides.
2. In a small bowl, crack an egg, then add the 1/2 cup cheddar cheese and stir to combine.
3. Pour 1/2 of the batter in the waffle maker and close the top.
4. Cooking for 3-4 minutes or until it reaches desired doneness.
5. Carefully remove from waffle maker and set aside for 2-3 minutes to give it time to crisp.
6. Follow the Directions again to make the second chaffle.

Nutrition:

- Calories: 122 kcal
- Fat: 9g
- Carbs: 5g
- Protein: 10g

2. <u>Cinnamon Keto Chaffles</u>

Preparation Time: 5 minutes

Cooking Time: 10 minutes

Servings: 3

Ingredients:

- 1/2 cup Mozzarella cheese
- 1 tablespoon almond flour
- 1/4 tsp. baking powder
- 1 egg
- 1 tsp. cinnamon
- 1 tsp. Granulated Swerve
- Cinnamon roll swirl Ingredients:
- 1 tbsp. butter
- 1 tsp. cinnamon
- 2 tsp. confectioner's swerve
- Keto Cinnamon Roll Glaze
- 1 tablespoon butter
- 1 tablespoon cream cheese
- 1/4 tsp. vanilla extract
- 2 tsp. swerve confectioners

Directions:

1. Plug in your Mini Dash Waffle maker and let it heat up.

2. In a small bowl mix the Mozzarella cheese, almond flour, baking powder, egg, 1 teaspoon cinnamon, and 1 teaspoon swerve granulated and set aside.
3. In another small bowl, add a tablespoon of butter, 1 teaspoon cinnamon, and 2 teaspoons of swerve confectioners' sweetener.
4. Microwave for 15 seconds and mix well.
5. Spray the waffle maker with nonstick spray and add 1/3 of the batter to your waffle maker. Swirl in 1/3 of the cinnamon, swerve, and butter mixture onto the top of it. Close the waffle maker and let cooking for 3-4 minutes.
6. When the first cinnamon roll chaffle is done, make the second and then make the third.
7. While the third chaffle is cooking place 1 tablespoon butter and 1 tablespoon of cream cheese in a small bowl. Heat in the microwave for 10-15 seconds. Start at 10, and if the cream cheese is not soft enough to mix with the butter heat for an additional 5 seconds.
8. Add the vanilla extract, and the swerve confectioner's sweetener to the butter and cream cheese and mix well using a whisk.
9. Drizzle keto cream cheese glaze on top of chaffle.

Nutrition:

- Calories: 370 kcal
- Fat: 26g
- Carbs: 5g
- Protein: 25g.

3. Broccoli & Cheese Chaffle

Preparation Time: 2 minutes

Cooking Time: 8 minutes

Servings: 2

Ingredients:

- 1/2 cup cheddar cheese
- 1/4 cup fresh chopped broccoli
- 1 egg
- 1/4 teaspoon garlic powder
- 1 tablespoon almond flour

Directions:

1. In a bowl, mix almond flour, cheddar cheese, egg, and garlic powder. I find it easiest to mix everything using a fork.
2. Add half the Broccoli and Cheese Chaffle batter to the Dish Mini waffle maker at a time.
3. Cooking chaffle batter in the waffle maker for 4 minutes.
4. Let each chaffle sit for 1-2 minutes on a plate to firm up. Enjoy alone or dipping in sour cream or ranch dressing.

Nutrition:

- Calories: 282 kcal
- Fat: 19,2g
- Carbs: 4g
- Protein: 19g.

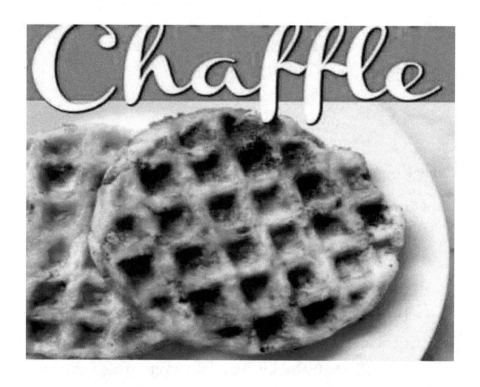

4. French Dip Chaffle Sandwich

Preparation Time: 5 minutes

Cooking Time: 12 minutes

Servings: 2

Ingredients:

- 1 egg white
- 1/4 cup Mozzarella cheese, shredded (packed)
- 1/4 cup sharp cheddar cheese, shredded (packed) 3/4 tsp. water
- 1 tsp. coconut flour
- 1/4 tsp. baking powder
- Pinch of salt

Directions:

1. Preheat oven to 425 degrees. Plug the Dash Mini Waffle Maker in the wall and grease lightly once it is hot.
2. Combine all of the ingredients in a bowl and stir to combine.
3. Spoon out 1/2 of the batter on the waffle maker and close lid. Set a timer for 4 minutes and do not lift the lid until the cooking time is complete. Lifting beforehand can cause the Chaffle keto sandwich recipe to separate and stick to the waffle iron. You have to let it cooking the entire 4 minutes before lifting the lid.

4. Remove the chaffle from the waffle iron and set aside. Repeat the same steps above with the rest of the chaffle batter.

5. Cover a cooking sheet with parchment paper and place chaffles a few inches apart.

6. Add 1/4 to 1/3 cup of the slow cooker keto roast beef from the following recipe. Make sure to drain the excess broth/gravy before adding to the top of the chaffle.

7. Add a slice of deli cheese or shredded cheese on top. Swiss and provolone are both great options. Place on the top rack of the oven for 5 minutes so that the cheese can melt. If you'd like the cheese to bubble and begin to brown, turn oven to broil for 1 min. (The swiss cheese may not brown) Enjoy open-faced with a small bowl of beef broth for dipping.

Nutrition:

- Calories: 510 kcal
- Fat: 35g
- Carbs: 2g
- Protein: 44g.

5. <u>Keto Chaffle Stuffing Recipe</u>

Preparation Time: 5 minutes

Cooking Time: 12 minutes

Servings: 4

Ingredients:

- Basic Chaffle ingredients:
- 1/2 cup cheese mozzarella, cheddar or a combo of both
- 2 eggs
- 1/4 tsp. garlic powder
- 1/2 tsp. onion powder
- 1/2 tsp. dried poultry seasoning
- 1/4 tsp. salt
- 1/4 tsp. pepper
- Stuffing ingredients:
- 1 small onion diced
- 2 celery stalks
- 4 oz. mushrooms diced
- 4 tbs butter for sauteing
- 3 eggs

Directions:

1. First, make your chaffles.
2. Preheat the mini waffle iron.
3. Preheat the oven to 350F
4. In a medium-size bowl, combine the chaffle ingredients.

5. Pour a 1/4 of the mixture into a mini waffle maker and cooking each chaffle for about 4 minutes each.
6. Once they are all cooked, set them aside.
7. In a small frying pan, sauté the onion, celery, and mushrooms until they are soft.
8. In a separate bowl, tear up the chaffles into small pieces, add the sauteed veggies, and 3 eggs. Mix until the ingredients are fully combined.
9. Add the stuffing mixture to a small casserole dish (about a 4 x 4) and bake it at 350 degrees for about 30 to 40 minutes.

Nutrition:

- Calories: 298 kcal
- Fat: 17g
- Carbs: 7,2
- Protein: 23g.

6. Chaffle Churros

Preparation Time: 10 min.

Cooking Time: 5 min.

Servings: 2

Ingredients:

- 1 egg
- 1 Tbsp. almond flour
- ½ tsp. vanilla extract
- 1 tsp. cinnamon, divided
- ¼ tsp. baking powder
- ½ cup shredded mozzarella
- 1 Tbsp. swerve confectioners' sugar substitute
- 1 Tbsp. swerve brown sugar substitute
- 1 Tbsp. butter, melted

Directions:

1. Turn on waffle maker to heat and oil it with cooking spray.
2. Mix egg, flour, vanilla extract, ½ tsp. cinnamon, baking powder, mozzarella, and sugar substitute in a bowl.
3. Place half of the mixture into waffle maker and cooking for 3-5 minutes, or until desired doneness. Remove and place the second half of the batter into the maker.
4. Cut chaffles into strips.
5. Place strips in a bowl and cover with melted butter.

6. Mix brown sugar substitute and the remaining cinnamon in a bowl. Pour sugar mixture over the strips and toss to coat them well.

Nutrition:

- Calories: 372 kcal
- Fat: 16g
- Carbs: 3g
- Protein: 40g.

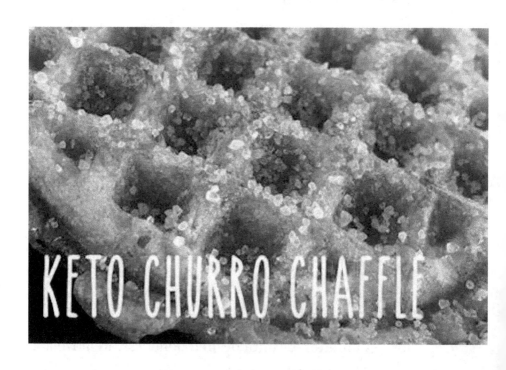

7. Cocoa Chaffles

Preparation Time: 5 min.

Cooking Time: 5 min.

Servings: 2

Ingredients:

- 1 egg
- 1½ Tbsp. unsweetened cocoa
- 2 Tbsp. lakanto monk fruit, or choice of sweetener
- 1 Tbsp. heavy cream
- 1 tsp. coconut flour
- ½ tsp. baking powder
- ½ tsp. vanilla
- For the Cheese Cream:
- 1 Tbsp. lakanto powdered sweetener
- 2 Tbsp. softened cream cheese
- ¼ tsp. vanilla

Directions:

1. Turn on waffle maker to heat and oil it with cooking spray. Combine all chaffle ingredients in a small bowl.
2. Pour one half of the chaffle mixture into waffle maker. Cooking for 3-5 minutes.
3. Remove and repeat with the second half if the mixture. Let chaffles sit for 2-3 to crisp up.

4. Combine all cream ingredients and spread on chaffle when they have cooled to room temperature.

Nutrition:

- Calories: 343 kcal
- Fat: 27g
- Carbs: 4g
- Protein: 21g

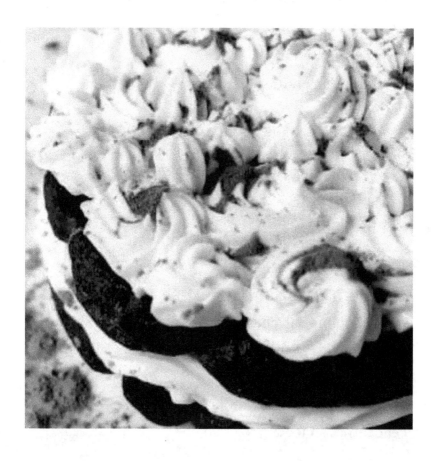

8. Crunchy Fish and Chaffle Bites

Cooking Time: 15 Minutes

Servings: 4

Ingredients:

- 1 lb. cod fillets, sliced into 4 slices
- 1 tsp. sea salt
- 1 tsp. garlic powder
- 1 egg, whisked
- 1 cup almond flour
- 2 tbsp. avocado oil
- Chaffle Ingredients:
- 2 eggs
- 1/2 cup cheddar cheese
- 2 tbsps. almond flour
- ½ tsp. Italian seasoning

Directions:

1. Mix together chaffle ingredients in a bowl and make 4 squares
2. Put the chaffles in a preheated chaffle maker.
3. Mix together the salt, pepper, and garlic powder in a mixing bowl. Toss the cod cubes in this mixture and let sit for 10 minutes.
4. Then dip each cod slice into the egg mixture and then into the almond flour.

5. Heat oil in skillet and fish cubes for about 2-3 minutes, until cooked and browned

6. Serve on chaffles and enjoy!

Nutrition:

- Calories: 173 kcal
- Fat: 10.4 g
- Fiber 8.5 g
- Carbs 15.3 g
- Protein: 5 g

SWEET CHAFFLE RECIPES

9. Belgium Chaffle

Preparation Time: 5 minutes

Cooking Time: 6 minutes

Serving: 1 regular Belgium chaffle

Ingredients:

- 1 cup grated cheddar cheese
- 2 eggs

Directions:

1. Preheat the waffle iron.
2. Beat the eggs then add the grated cheddar cheese.
3. Make sure that the mixture is well combined.
4. Cook the mixture for about six minutes.

Nutrition:

- for 1 chaffle Calories: 460 kcal
- Cholesterol: 490 mg
- Carbohydrates: 2 g
- Protein: 44 g
- Fat: 33 g

10. French Toast Chaffle

Preparation Time: 5 minutes

Cooking Time: 10 minutes

Serving: 2 mini chaffles

Ingredients:

- 1 egg
- ½ cup grated mozzarella cheese
- 2 tbsp almond flour, ALLERGY WARNING
- 1 tsp vanilla extract
- 1 tsp cinnamon
- 1 tsp granulated sweetener of choice

Directions:

1. Preheat your waffle iron.
2. Mix all the chaffle ingredients well.
3. Use half of the mixture and cook the chaffle for about five minutes.
4. Add an extra minute to the cooking if you want a crispier chaffle.
5. Repeat until all the batter is used.
6. Add some sugar-free cinnamon syrup and enjoy these chaffles still warm.

Nutrition:

- for 1 mini chaffle Calories: 180 kcal
- Carbohydrates: 7 g
- Protein: 11 g
- Fat: 12 g

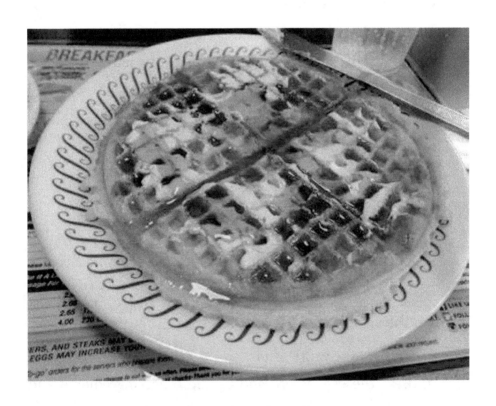

11. Banana Nut Chaffle Recipe

Preparation Time: 3 minutes

Cooking Time: 8 minutes

Serving: 2 mini chaffles

Ingredients:

- 1 egg
- ¼ tsp vanilla extract
- ¼ tsp banana extract
- 1 tbsp cream cheese, room temperature, and softened
- ½ cup grated mozzarella cheese
- 1 tbsp monk fruit confectioners, or confectioner's sweetener of choice
- 1 tbsp sugar-free cheesecake pudding, optional
- Toppings:
- Pecans
- Sugar-free caramel sauce. or keto-safe sauce of preference

Directions:

1. Preheat the waffle iron.
2. Beat the egg before adding the other ingredients and make sure that everything is coated in the egg mixture.
3. Use half of the batter and cook for about four minutes.
4. Remove chaffle to rest while cooking the second mini chaffle.

5. This chaffle can be enjoyed warm with suggested toppings or toppings of your own choice. Enjoy.

Nutrition:

- for 1 mini chaffle Calories: 119 kcal
- Cholesterol: 111 mg
- Carbohydrates: 2.7 g
- Protein: 8.8 g
- Fat: 7.8 g
- Sugar: 1.1 g

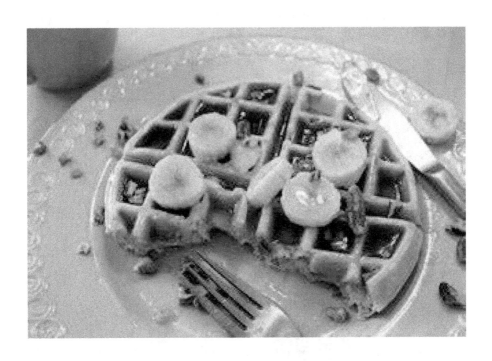

12. Banana Foster Chaffle Pancakes

Preparation Time: 5 minutes

Cooking Time: 20 minutes

Serving: 4 regular chaffles

Ingredients:

- 4 large eggs
- 1 cup almond flour, ALLERGY WARNING
- ⅓ cup flaxseed meal
- 1 tsp vanilla extract
- ½ medium banana, slightly overripe
- 4 oz cream cheese
- 2 tsp baking powder
- ½ tsp banana extract, optional
- Liquid stevia or sweetener of choice, optional
- Ingredients for Banana Foster Topping:
- 8 tbsp salted butter
- ½ tsp cinnamon
- ½ tsp vanilla extract
- ½ tsp banana extract
- ¼ cup sugar-free maple syrup
- ½ cup brown sugar substitute or granulated sweetener with maple extract
- ½ medium banana, sliced into discs
- ⅛–¼ tsp xanthan gum, optional
- 2 tbsp dark rum or bourbon, optional
- ¼ cup pecans chopped, optional

Directions:

1. Preheat the waffle iron or skillet.

2. Add all the chaffle ingredients to a blender and blend until smooth.
3. Add ¼ of the batter to the waffle iron and cook for about two–three minutes, add an extra minute to cooking if the chaffle isn't set.
4. Repeat until all the batter is used.
5. Directions of Topping:
6. At a medium temperature combine the banana extract, rum or bourbon, butter, and vanilla in a skillet.
7. As the mixture starts to bubble, add the sliced bananas in a single layer and allow them to cook for between two to three minutes. Do not stir.
8. After the time has passed, add the cinnamon, brown sugar substitute, and sugar-free maple syrup.
9. Stir and let the mixture simmer until all the brown sugar substitute has become melted and incorporated into the butter.
10. If the brown sugar substitute isn't blending with the butter, then add the xanthan gum to the simmering mixture. This will also help to thicken up the sauce.
11. Depending on your preference, you can either add the pecans to the simmering sauce or add it after pouring the source on the chaffles.
12. Add the warm sauce to the cooled chaffles.

13. Add a scoop or two of keto-friendly ice cream to make a unique taste experience. Or simply enjoy the chaffle with no sauce.

Nutrition:

- for two regular chaffle with 2 ½ tbsp of topping Calories: 417 kcal
- Cholesterol: 170 mg
- Carbohydrates: 13 g
- Fat: 37 g
- Sugar: 7 g
- Protein: 10 g

13. Chocolate Chip Chaffles

Preparation Time: 3 minutes

Cooking Time: 8 minutes

Serving: 2 mini chaffles

Ingredients:

- ½ cup grated mozzarella cheese
- ½ tbsp granulated Swerve, or sweetener of choice
- 1 tbsp almond flour, ALLERGY WARNING
- 2 tbsp low carb, sugar-free chocolate chips
- 1 egg
- ¼ tsp cinnamon

Directions:

1. Preheat your waffle iron.
2. In a bowl, mix the almond flour, egg, cinnamon, mozzarella cheese, Swerve, chocolate chips.
3. Place half the batter in the waffle iron and cook for four minutes.
4. Remove chaffle and cook the remaining batter.
5. Let chaffles cool before serving.
6. Enjoy these chaffles with some keto-safe chocolate sauce and some whipped cream.

Nutrition:

- for 1 mini chaffle Calories: 136 kcal
- Cholesterol: 104 mg
- Carbohydrates: 2 g
- Protein: 10 g
- Fat: 10 g
- Sugar: 1 g

14. Chocolate Chaffle

Preparation Time: 3 minutes

Cooking Time: 5 minutes

Serving: 1 chaffle, 2 mini chaffles

Ingredients:

- 1 tsp vanilla extract
- 1 tbsp cocoa powder, unsweetened.
- 1 egg
- 2 tbsp almond flour, Allergy Warning
- 2 tsp monk fruit
- 1 oz cream cheese

Directions:

1. Preheat the waffle iron.
2. Soften the cream cheese then whisk together the other ingredients well.
3. Pour the batter into the center of the waffle iron and spread out.
4. Cook batter for between three and five minutes.
5. Remove chaffle once set and serve.
6. Consider making your own keto-friendly ice cream to go with this treat so that you can enjoy it while it is still warm.

Nutrition:

- for 1 regular chaffle Calories: 261 kcal
- Carbohydrates: 4 g
- Protein: 11.5 g
- Fat: 22.2 g

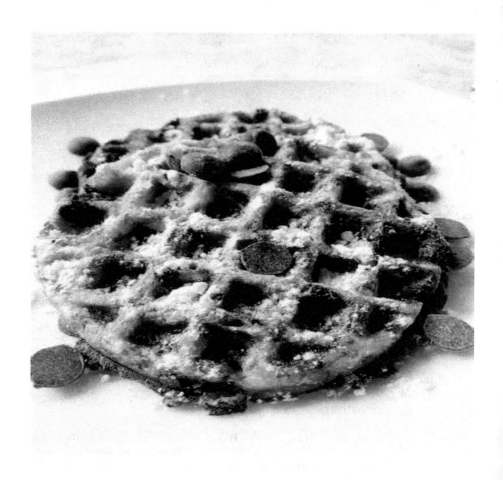

15. Basic Sweet Keto Chaffles

Preparation Time: 5 minutes

Cooking Time: 5 Minutes

Servings: 2

Ingredients:

- 1 egg
- ½ cup shredded Cheddar cheese

Directions:

1. Turn on waffle maker to heat and oil it with cooking spray.
2. Whisk egg in a bowl until well beaten.
3. Add cheese to the egg and stir well to combine.
4. Pour ½ batter into the waffle maker and close the top. Cooking for 3-5 minutes.
5. Transfer chaffle to a plate and set aside for 2-3 minutes to crisp up.
6. Repeat for remaining batter.

Nutrition:

- Calories: 127 kcal
- Fat: 5 g
- Carbs: 1 g
- Protein: 20 g

16. Mayonnaise Chaffle

Preparation Time: 5 minutes

Cooking Time: 10 Minutes

Servings: 3

Ingredients:

- 1 large organic egg, beaten1 tablespoon mayonnaise
- 2 tablespoons almond flour
- 1/8 teaspoon organic baking powder
- 1 teaspoon water2–4 drops liquid stevia

Directions:

1. Preheat a mini waffle iron and then grease it.
2. In a medium bowl, put all ingredients and with a fork, mix until well combined. Place half of the mixture into preheated waffle iron and cooking for about 4–5 minutes.
3. Repeat with the remaining mixture.
4. Serve warm.

Nutrition:

- Calories: 208 kcal
- Fat: 7 g
- Carbs: 22 g
- Protein: 19 g

SAVORY CHAFFLE RECIPES

17. Basil Chaffles

Preparation Time: 10 minutes

Cooking Time: 16 minutes

Servings: 3Ingredients:

Ingredients:

- 2 organic eggs, beaten
- ½ cup Mozzarella cheese, shredded
- 1 tablespoon Parmesan cheese, grated
- 1 teaspoon dried basil, crushed
- Pinch of salt

Directions:

1. Preheat a mini waffle iron and then grease it.
2. In a medium bowl, place all ingredients and mix until well combined.
3. Place 1/3 of the mixture into preheated waffle iron and cooking for about 3-4 minutes or until golden brown.
4. Repeat with the remaining mixture.
5. Serve warm.

Nutrition:

- Calories: 212 kcal
- Total Fat: 3.8g
- Saturated Fat: 0.7g
- Cholesterol: 29mg
- Sodium: 329mg
- Carbohydrate: 29g
- Dietary Fiber: 1.4g
- Sugars: 0.9g
- Protein: 14.9g
- Calcium: 37mg
- Phosphorous: 361 mg
- Potassium: 171mg

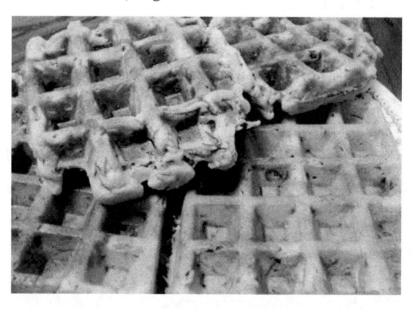

18. Sage & Coconut Milk Chaffles

Preparation Time: 10 minutes

Cooking Time: 24 minutes

Servings: 6

Ingredients:

- ¾ cup coconut flour, sifted
- 1½ teaspoons organic baking powder
- ½ teaspoon dried ground sage
- 1/8 teaspoon garlic powder
- 1/8 teaspoon salt
- 1 organic egg
- 1 cup unsweetened coconut milk
- ¼ cup water
- 1½ tablespoons coconut oil, melted
- ½ cup cheddar cheese, shredded

Directions:

1. Preheat a waffle iron and then grease it.
2. In a bowl, add the flour, baking powder, sage, garlic powder and salt and mix well.
3. Add the egg, coconut milk, water and coconut oil and mix until a stiff mixture form.
4. Add the cheese and gently stir to combine.
5. Divide the mixture into 6 portions.

6. Place 1 portion of the mixture into preheated waffle iron and cooking for about 4 minutes or until golden brown.
7. Repeat with the remaining mixture.
8. Serve warm.

Nutrition:

- Calories: 579 kcal
- Fat: 18 g
- Carbs: 33 g
- Protein: 11 g

19. Dried Herbs Chaffles

Preparation Time: 5 minutes

Cooking Time: 8 minutes

Servings: 2

Ingredients:

- 1 organic egg, beaten
- ½ cup Cheddar cheese, shredded
- 1 tablespoon almond flour
- Pinch of dried thyme, crushed
- Pinch of dried rosemary, crushed

Directions:

1. Preheat a mini waffle iron and then grease it.
2. In a bowl, place all the ingredients and beat until well combined.
3. Place half of the mixture into preheated waffle iron and cooking for about 3-4 minutes or until golden brown.
4. Repeat with the remaining mixture.
5. Serve warm.

Nutrition:

- Calories: 245 kcal
- Fat: 7 g
- Carbs 23 g
- Protein: 10 g

20. 3-Cheeses Herbed Chaffles

Preparation Time: 10 minutes

Cooking Time: 12 minutes

Servings: 4

Ingredients:

- 4 tablespoons almond flour
- 1 tablespoon coconut flour
- 1 teaspoon mixed dried herbs
- ½ teaspoon organic baking powder
- ¼ teaspoon garlic powder
- ¼ teaspoon onion powder
- Salt and freshly ground black pepper, to taste
- ¼ cup cream cheese, softened
- 3 large organic eggs
- ½ cup Cheddar cheese, grated
- 1/3 cup Parmesan cheese, grated

Directions:

1. Preheat a waffle iron and then grease it.
2. In a bowl, mix together the flours, dried herbs, baking powder and seasoning and mix well.
3. In a separate bowl, put cream cheese and eggs and beat until well combined.
4. Add the flour mixture, cheddar and Parmesan cheese and mix until well combined.

5. Place the desired amount of the mixture into preheated waffle iron and cooking for about 2-3 minutes or until golden brown.
6. Repeat with the remaining mixture.
7. Serve warm.

Nutrition:

- Calories: 579 kcal
- Fat: 18 g
- Carbs: 33 g
- Protein: 11 g

21. Italian Inspired Chaffles

Preparation Time: 10 minutes

Cooking Time: 8 minutes

Servings: 2

Ingredients:

- ½ cup Mozzarella cheese, shredded
- 1 tablespoon Parmesan cheese, shredded
- 1 organic egg
- ¾ teaspoon coconut flour
- ¼ teaspoon organic baking powder
- 1/8 teaspoon Italian seasoning
- Pinch of salt

Directions:

1. Preheat a mini waffle iron and then grease it.
2. In a medium bowl, place all ingredients and with a fork, mix until well combined.
3. Place half of the mixture into preheated waffle iron and cooking for about 3-4 minutes or until golden brown.
4. Repeat with the remaining mixture.
5. Serve warm.

Nutrition:

- Calories: 221 kcal
- Fat: 19g
- Carb: 3g
- Phosphorus: 119mg
- Potassium: 140mg
- Sodium: 193mg
- Protein: 8g

22. Garlic Herb Blend Chaffles

Preparation Time: 10 minutes

Cooking Time: 8 minutes

Servings: 2

Ingredients:

- 1 large organic egg, beaten
- ¼ cup Parmesan cheese, shredded
- ¼ cup Mozzarella cheese, shredded
- ½ tablespoon butter, melted
- 1 teaspoon garlic herb blend seasoning
- Salt, to taste

Directions:

1. Preheat a mini waffle iron and then grease it.
2. In a bowl, place all the ingredients and beat until well combined.
3. Place half of the mixture into preheated waffle iron and cooking for about 3-4 minutes or until golden brown.
4. Repeat with the remaining mixture.
5. Serve warm.

Nutrition:

- Calories: 208 kcal
- Fat: 7 g
- Carbs: 22 g
- Protein: 19 g

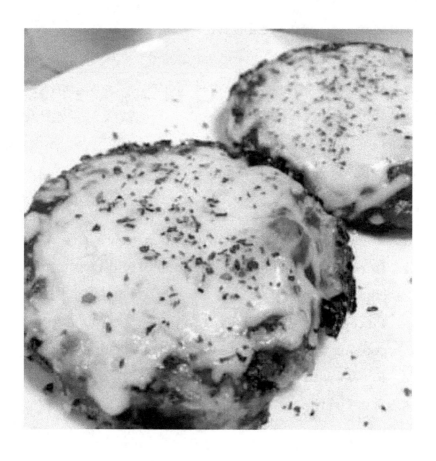

23. BBQ Rub Chaffles

Preparation Time: 5 minutes

Cooking Time: 20 minutes

Servings: 4

Ingredients:

- 2 organic eggs, beaten
- 1 cup Cheddar cheese, shredded
- ½ teaspoon BBQ rub
- ¼ teaspoon organic baking powder

Directions:

1. Preheat a mini waffle iron and then grease it.
2. In a medium bowl, place all ingredients and with a fork, mix until well combined.
3. Place ¼ of the mixture into preheated waffle iron and cooking for about 5 minutes or until golden brown.
4. Repeat with the remaining mixture.
5. Serve warm.

Nutrition:

- Calories: 186 kcal
- Carbohydrate: 43.7 g
- Sodium: 130 mg
- Potassium: 135 mg
- Phosphorus: 18 mg
- Dietary Fiber: 2.4 g
- Fat: 2.3 g
- Protein: 2.28 g

24. Bagel Seasoning Chaffles

Preparation Time: 10 minutes

Cooking Time: 20 minutes

Servings: 4

Ingredients:

- 1 large organic egg
- 1 cup Mozzarella cheese, shredded
- 1 tablespoon almond flour
- 1 teaspoon organic baking powder
- 2 teaspoons bagel seasoning
- ¼ teaspoon garlic powder
- ¼ teaspoon onion powder

Directions:

1. Preheat a mini waffle iron and then grease it.
2. In a medium bowl, place all ingredients and with a fork, mix until well combined.
3. Place ¼ of the mixture into preheated waffle iron and cooking for about 3-4 minutes or until golden brown.
4. Repeat with the remaining mixture.
5. Serve warm.

Nutrition:

- Calories: 208 kcal
- Fat: 7g
- Carbs 22 g
- Protein: 19 g

VEGETARIAN CHAFFLE RECIPES

25. Crispy Bagel Chaffles

Preparation Time: 5 minutes

Cooking Time: 30 Minutes

Servings: 2

Ingredients:

- 2 eggs
- ½ cup parmesan cheese
- 1 tsp bagel seasoning
- ½ cup mozzarella cheese
- 2 teaspoons almond flour

Directions:

1. Turn on waffle maker to heat and oil it with cooking spray.
2. Evenly sprinkle half of cheeses to a griddle and let them melt. Then toast for 30 seconds and leave them wait for batter.
3. Whisk eggs, other half of cheeses, almond flour, and bagel seasoning in a small bowl.
4. Pour batter into the waffle maker. Cook for minutes.
5. Let cool for 2-3 minutes before serving.

Nutrition:

- Calories: 117 kcal
- Fat: 2.1g
- Carbs 18.2g
- Protein: 22.7g
- Potassium: (K) 296mg
- Sodium: (Na) 81mg
- Phosphorous: 28 mg

26. Cinnamon Chaffle Rolls

Preparation Time: 7 minutes

Cooking Time: 10 Minutes

Servings: 2

Ingredients:

- 1/2 cup mozzarella cheese
- 1 tbsp. almond flour
- 1 egg
- 1 tsp cinnamon
- 1 tsp stevia
- Cinnamon Roll Glaze
- 1 tbsp. butter
- 1 tbsp. cream cheese
- 1 tsp. cinnamon
- 1/4 tsp vanilla extract
- 1 tbsp. coconut flour

Directions:

1. Switch on a round waffle maker and let it heat up.
2. In a small bowl mix together cheese, egg, flour, cinnamon powder, and stevia in a bowl.
3. Spray the round waffle maker with nonstick spray.
4. Pour the batter in a waffle maker and close the lid.
5. Close the waffle maker and cook for about 3-4 minutes Utes.

6. Once chaffles are cooked, remove from Maker
7. Mix together butter, cream cheese, cinnamon, vanilla and coconut flour in a bowl.
8. Spread this glaze over chaffle and roll up.
9. Serve and enjoy!

Nutrition:

- Calories: 176 kcal
- Fat: 2.1g
- Carbs: 27g
- Protein: 15.1g
- Potassium: (K) 242mg
- Sodium: (Na) 72mg
- Phosphorous: 555.3 mg

27. Broccoli & Almond Flour Chaffles

Preparation Time: 6 minutes

Cooking Time: 8 Minutes

Servings: 2

Ingredients:

- 1 organic egg, beaten
- ½ cup Cheddar cheese, shredded
- ¼ cup fresh broccoli, chopped
- 1 tablespoon almond flour
- ¼ teaspoon garlic powder

Directions:

1. Preheat a mini waffle iron and then grease it.
2. In a bowl, place all ingredients and mix until well combined.
3. Place half of the mixture into preheated waffle iron and cook for about 4 minutes or until golden brown.
4. Repeat with the remaining mixture.
5. Serve warm.

Nutrition:

- Calories: 221 kcal
- Protein: 17 g
- Carbs: 31 g
- Fat: 8 g
- Sodium: (Na) 235 mg
- Potassium: (K) 176 mg
- Phosphorus: 189 mg

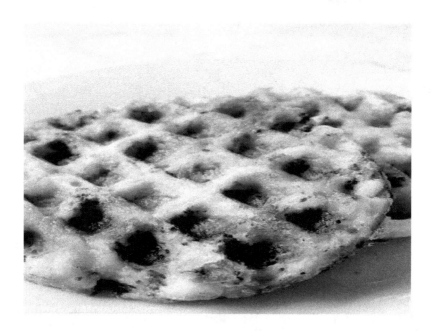

28. Cheddar Jalapeño Chaffle

Preparation Time: 6 minutes

Cooking Time: 5 Minutes

Servings: 2

Ingredients:

- 2 large eggs
- ½ cup shredded mozzarella
- ¼ cup almond flour
- ½ tsp baking powder
- ¼ cup shredded cheddar cheese
- 2 Tbsp diced jalapeños jarred or canned
- For the toppings:
- ½ cooked bacon, chopped
- 2 Tbsp cream cheese
- ¼ jalapeño slices

Directions:

1. Turn on waffle maker to heat and oil it with cooking spray.
2. Mix mozzarella, eggs, baking powder, almond flour, and garlic powder in a bowl.
3. Sprinkle 2 Tbsp cheddar cheese in a thin layer on waffle maker, and ½ jalapeño.
4. Ladle half of the egg mixture on top of the cheese and jalapeños.

5. Cook for minutes, or until done.

6. Repeat for the second chaffle.

7. Top with cream cheese, bacon, and jalapeño slices.

Nutrition:

- Calories: 221 kcal
- Protein: 13 g
- Carbs 1 g
- Fat: 34 g
- Sodium: (Na) 80 mg
- Potassium: (K) 119 mg
- Phosphorus: 158 mg

29. Spinach & Cauliflower Chaffles

Preparation Time: 6 minutes

Cooking Time: 10 Minutes

Servings: 2

Ingredients:

- ½ cup frozen chopped spinach, thawed and squeezed
- ½ cup cauliflower, chopped finely
- ½ cup Cheddar cheese, shredded
- ½ cup Mozzarella cheese, shredded
- 1/3 cup Parmesan cheese, shredded
- 2 organic eggs
- 1 tablespoon butter, melted
- 1 teaspoon garlic powder
- 1 teaspoon onion powder
- Salt and freshly ground black pepper, to taste

Directions:

1. Preheat a waffle iron and then grease it.
2. In a medium bowl, place all ingredients and, mix until well combined.
3. Place half of the mixture into preheated waffle iron and cook for about 4-5 minutes or until golden brown.
4. Repeat with the remaining mixture.
5. Serve warm.

Nutrition:

- Calories: 221 kcal
- Protein: 11 g
- Carbs 26 g
- Fat: 7 g
- Sodium: (Na) 143 mg
- Potassium: (K)197 mg
- Phosphorus: 182 mg

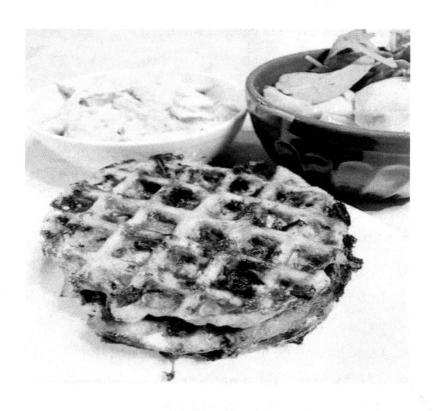

30. Rosemary in Chaffles

Preparation Time: 6 minutes

Cooking Time: 8 Minutes

Servings: 2

Ingredients:

- 1 organic egg, beaten
- ½ cup Cheddar cheese, shredded
- 1 tablespoon almond flour
- 1 tablespoon fresh rosemary, chopped
- Pinch of salt and freshly ground black pepper

Directions:

1. Preheat a mini waffle iron and then grease it.
2. For chaffles: In a medium bowl, place all ingredients and with a fork, mix until well combined.
3. Place half of the mixture into preheated waffle iron and cook for about 4 minutes or until golden brown.
4. Repeat with the remaining mixture.
5. Serve warm.

Nutrition:

- Calories: 221 kcal
- Protein: 12 g
- Carbs 29 g
- Fat: 8 g
- Sodium: (Na) 398 mg
- Potassium: (K) 347 mg
- Phosphorus: 241 mg

31. Zucchini Chaffles With Peanut Butter

Preparation Time: 5 minutes

Cooking Time: 5 Minutes

Servings: 2

Ingredients:

- 1 cup zucchini grated
- 1 egg beaten
- 1/2 cup shredded parmesan cheese
- 1/4 cup shredded mozzarella cheese
- 1 tsp dried basil
- 1/2 tsp. salt
- 1/2 tsp. black pepper
- 2 tbsps. peanut butter for topping

Directions:

1. Sprinkle salt over zucchini and let it sit for minutes Utes.
2. Squeeze out water from zucchini.
3. Beat egg with zucchini, basil. salt mozzarella cheese, and pepper.
4. Sprinkle ½ of the parmesan cheese over preheated waffle maker and pour zucchini batter over it.
5. Sprinkle the remaining cheese over it.
6. Close the lid.
7. Cook zucchini chaffles for about 4-8 minutes Utes.

8. Remove chaffles from the maker and repeat with the remaining batter.

9. Serve with peanut butter on top and enjoy!

Nutrition:

- Calories: 124 kcal
- Protein: 15 g
- Carbs 0 g
- Fat: 7 g
- Sodium: (Na) 161 mg
- Potassium: (K) 251 mg
- Phosphorus: 220 mg

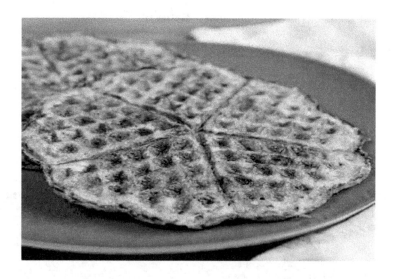

32. Zucchini in Chaffles

Preparation Time: 10 minutes

Cooking Time: 18 Minutes

Servings: 2

Ingredients:

- 2 large zucchinis, grated and squeezed
- 2 large organic eggs
- 2/3 cup Cheddar cheese, shredded
- 2 tablespoons coconut flour
- ½ teaspoon garlic powder
- ½ teaspoon red pepper flakes, crushed
- Salt, to taste

Directions:

1. Preheat a waffle iron and then grease it.
2. In a medium bowl, place all ingredients and, mix until well combined.
3. Place ¼ of the mixture into preheated waffle iron and cook for about 4-4½ minutes or until golden brown.
4. Repeat with the remaining mixture.
5. Serve warm.

Nutrition:

- Calories: 311 kcal
- Protein: 16 g
- Carbs 17 g
- Fat: 15 g
- Sodium: (Na) 31 mg
- Potassium: (K) 418 mg
- Phosphorus: 257 mg

SPECIAL CHAFFLE RECIPES

33. Christmas Smoothie with Chaffles

Preparation Time: 10 minutes

Cooking Time: 0 Minutes

Servings: 2

Ingredients:

- 1 cup coconut milk
- 2 tbsps. almonds chopped
- ¼ cup cherries
- 1 pinch sea salt
- 1/4 cup ice cubes
- For Topping
- 2 oz. keto chocolate chips
- 2 oz. cherries
- 2 minutes chaffles
- 2 scoop heavy cream, frozen

Directions:

1. Add almond milk, almonds, cherries, salt and ice in a blender, blend for 2 minutes Utes until smooth and fluffy.
2. Pour the smoothie into glasses.

3. Top with one scoop heavy cream, chocolate chips, cherries and chaffle in each glass.

4. Serve and enjoy!

Nutrition:

- Calories: 106.58 kcal
- Carbohydrate: 8.20 g
- Protein: 4.77 g
- Sodium: 51.91 mg
- Potassium: 87.83 mg
- Phosphorus: 49.41 mg
- Dietary Fiber: 0.58 g
- Fat: 5 g

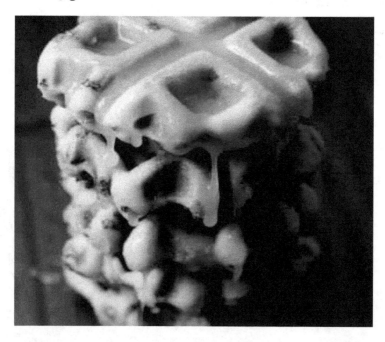

34. Raspberry and Chocolate Chaffle

Preparation Time: 5 minutes

Cooking Time: 7–9 Minutes

Servings: 2

Ingredients:

- Batter
- 4 eggs
- 2 ounces cream cheese, softened
- 2 ounces sour cream
- 1 teaspoon vanilla extract
- 5 tablespoons almond flour
- ¼ cup cocoa powder
- 1½ teaspoons baking powder
- 2 ounces fresh or frozen raspberries
- Other
- 2 tablespoons butter to brush the waffle maker
- Fresh sprigs of mint to garnish

Directions:

1. Preheat the waffle maker.
2. Add the eggs, cream cheese and sour cream to a bowl and stir with a wire whisk until just combined.
3. Add the vanilla extract and mix until combined.
4. Stir in the almond flour, cocoa powder, and baking powder and mix until combined.

5. Add the raspberries and stir until combined.

6. Brush the heated waffle maker with butter and add a few tablespoons of the batter.

7. Close the lid and cook for about 8 minutes depending on your waffle maker.

8. Serve with fresh sprigs of mint.

Nutrition:

- Calories: 186 kcal
- Carbohydrate: 43.7 g
- Sodium: 130 mg
- Potassium: 135 mg
- Phosphorus: 18 mg
- Dietary Fiber: 2.4 g
- Fat: 2.3 g
- Protein: 2.28 g

35. Keto Belgian Sugar Chaffles

Preparation Time: 8 minutes

Cooking Time: 24 Minutes

Servings: 2

Ingredients:

- 1 egg, beaten
- 2 tbsp swerve brown sugar
- ½ tbsp butter, melted
- 1 tsp vanilla extract
- 1 cup finely grated Parmesan cheese

Directions:

1. Preheat the waffle iron.
2. Mix all the ingredients in a medium bowl.
3. Open the iron and pour in a quarter of the mixture. Close and cook until crispy, 6 minutes.
4. Remove the chaffle onto a plate and make 3 more with the remaining ingredients.
5. Cut each chaffle into wedges, plate, allow cooling and serve.

Nutrition:

- Calories: 220 kcal
- Carbohydrate: 2.59 g
- Sodium: 88 mg
- Potassium: 133.5 mg
- Phosphorus: 68.5 mg
- Dietary Fiber: 1.7 g
- Fat: 23.7 g
- Protein: 3.2 g

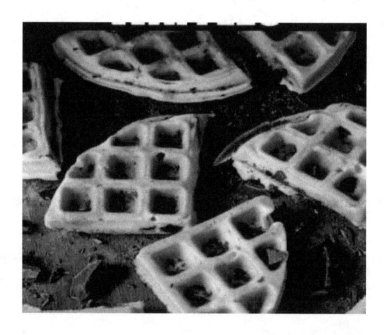

36. Pumpkin Chaffle Plus Maple Syrup

Preparation Time: 10 minutes

Cooking Time: 16 Minutes

Servings: 2

Ingredients:

- 2 eggs, beaten
- ½ cup mozzarella cheese, shredded
- 1 teaspoon coconut flour
- ¾ teaspoon baking powder
- ¾ teaspoon pumpkin pie spice
- 2 teaspoons pureed pumpkin
- 4 teaspoons heavy whipping cream
- ½ teaspoon vanilla
- Pinch salt
- 2 teaspoons maple syrup (sugar-free)

Directions:

1. Turn your waffle maker on.
2. Mix all the ingredients except maple syrup in a large bowl.
3. Pour half of the batter into the waffle maker.
4. Close and cook for minutes.
5. Transfer to a plate to cool for 2 minutes.
6. Repeat the steps with the remaining mixture.

7. Drizzle the maple syrup on top of the chaffles before serving.

Nutrition:

- Calories: 183 kcal
- Carbohydrate: 17.9 g
- Protein: 0.3 g
- Sodium: 2 g
- Potassium: 100 mg
- Phosphorus: 12.5 mg
- Dietary Fiber: 1.4 g
- Fat: 14.17 g

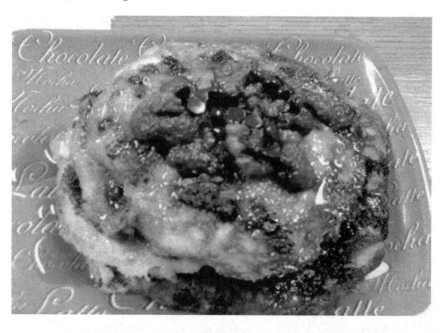

37. <u>Maple Syrup and Vanilla Chaffle</u>

Preparation Time: 6 minutes

Cooking Time: 12 Minutes

Servings: 2

Ingredients:

- 1 egg, beaten
- ¼ cup mozzarella cheese, shredded
- 1 oz. cream cheese
- 1 teaspoon vanilla
- 1 tablespoon keto maple syrup
- 1 teaspoon sweetener
- 1 teaspoon baking powder
- 4 tablespoons almond flour

Directions:

1. Preheat your waffle maker.
2. Add all the ingredients to a bowl.
3. Mix well.
4. Pour some of the batter into the waffle maker.
5. Cover and cook for 4 minutes.
6. Transfer chaffle to a plate and let cool for 2 minutes.
7. Repeat the same process with the remaining mixture.

Nutrition:

- Calories: 74 kcal
- Carbohydrate: 0.1 g
- Protein: 7 g
- Sodium: 121.9 g
- Potassium: 89.5 mg
- Phosphorus: 75 mg
- Dietary Fiber: 0 g
- Fat: 5.16 g

38. Sweet Vanilla Chocolate Chaffle

Preparation Time: 10 minutes

Cooking Time: 10 Minutes

Servings: 2

Ingredients:

- 1 egg, lightly beaten
- 1/4 tsp cinnamon
- 1/2 tsp vanilla
- 1 tbsp Swerve
- 2 tsp unsweetened cocoa powder
- 1 tbsp coconut flour
- 2 oz cream cheese, softened

Directions:

1. Add all ingredients into the small bowl and mix until well combined.
2. Spray waffle maker with cooking spray.
3. Pour batter in the hot waffle maker and cook until golden brown.
4. Serve and enjoy.

Nutrition:

- Calories: 278.5 kcal
- Carbohydrate: 38.72 g
- Protein: 1.3 g
- Sodium: 76.33 mg
- Potassium: 229.1 mg
- Phosphorus: 59.2 mg
- Dietary Fiber: 7.4 g
- Fat: 6 g

39. Thanksgiving Keto Chaffles

Servings: 5

Cooking Time: 15minutes

Servings: 2

Ingredients:

- 4 oz. cheese, shredded
- 5 eggs
- 1 tsp. stevia
- 1 tsp baking powder
- 2 tsp vanilla extract
- 1/4 cup almond butter, melted
- 3 tbsps. almond milk
- 1 tsp avocado oil for greasing

Directions:

1. Crack eggs in a small mixing bowl; mix the eggs, almond flour, stevia, and baking powder.
2. Add the melted butter slowly to the flour mixture, mix well to ensure a smooth consistency.
3. Add the almond milk and vanilla to the flour and butter mixture, be sure to mix well.
4. Preheat waffles maker according to the manufacturer's instruction and grease it with avocado oil.
5. Pour the mixture into the waffle maker and cook until golden brown.

6. Dust coconut flour on chaffles and serve with coconut cream on the top.

Nutrition:

- Calories: 165 kcal
- Carbohydrate: 3.8 g
- Protein: 9.2 g
- Sodium: 797 mg
- Potassium: 193 mg
- Phosphorus: 202.5 mg
- Dietary Fiber: 0.7 g
- Fat: 15.22 g

40. Garlic Cauliflower Chaffle

Preparation Time: 10 minutes

Cooking Time: 8 Minutes

Servings: 2

Ingredients:

- 1 egg, beaten
- 1 cup cauliflower rice
- ½ cup cheddar cheese, shredded
- 1 teaspoon garlic powder

Directions:

1. Plug in your waffle maker.
2. Mix all the ingredients in a bowl.
3. Transfer half of the mixture to the waffle maker.
4. Close the device and cook for minutes.
5. Put the chaffle on a plate to cool for 2 minutes.
6. Repeat procedure to make the next chaffle.

Nutrition:

- Calories: 212 kcal
- Total Fat: 3.8g
- Saturated Fat: 0.7g
- Cholesterol: 29mg

- Sodium: 329mg
- Carbohydrate: 29g
- Dietary Fiber: 1.4g
- Sugars: 0.9g
- Protein: 14.9g
- Calcium: 37mg
- Phosphorous: 361 mg
- Potassium: 171mg

CONCLUSION

Chaffles is the amazing new invention you've been waiting for. It's a revolutionary, patent-pending, and 100% vegan protein bar with a thousand uses.

What are chaffles? Chaffles is a delicious new product that can be used to replace the high fat and high sugar snacks in your diet like cheese chips or chocolate bars. It's also gluten-free, vegan, non-GMO, low in sodium and preservative free! The best part is that chaffles taste just as good as candy! You'll never want anything else again after trying this life changing snack.

The combination of protein and savory chaffle taste will keep you wanting to eat more every time. Chaffles are also a great substitute for those times that you feel like having something sweet, but want something healthy with a lot of flavor.

Chaffles come in an assortment of flavors like Pecan Pie or Cherry Pie and can be served with a drizzle of your favorite nut butter or cinnamon sugar for an awesome snack. Or you can create your own combinations by mixing them up the way that makes your mouth water.

Chaffles are great for both kids and adults. They're the perfect snack to bring on a hike for an afternoon treat or to eat on a road trip or flights. Even better, they create a new way for parents to get their kids to eat protein without them even knowing what they're eating. Now if you want your children to enjoy healthy food without complaining, chaffles will be your best friend.

No matter what you eat chaffles with, it will never disappoint! Have it with chicken noodle soup or mashed potatoes for dinner or have it with salad at lunch.

Chaffle is a perfect combination for keto dieters. Besides, keto diet is always low in carbs and high in fat so chaffle is an amazing option for it.

Chaffles are very versatile and can be used as a spread for your favorite bagel or toast, or even on top of a pizza before baking it. You can also use chaffles as an ingredient for your own meals like pancakes, pies, donuts, breads and so much more!

Chaffle comes in two different flavors: savory and sweet. The savory flavor is more of a BBQ flavor while the sweet flavor is more cookie dough style. The savory chaffles are perfect for replacing things like bread and crackers, while sweet chaffles can be used as a dessert or drink! You can also add chaffle to your favorite dessert recipes for an amazing taste.

Chaffles are the most unique tasting protein bar around that is also good for you. You won't believe how good they taste until you try them for yourself. This incredible product is sure to revolutionize your snacking experience and change the way you think about eating healthy forever.

Always remember when making your own chaffle recipes, you can choose from almost any combination of things like fruits, cereals, nuts and seeds. You can even use different types of chocolate in some recipes. Anything goes with chaffle!

What's even more exciting is that chaffles come in many sizes to fit anyone's taste and diet.

It's time to ditch your unhealthy snacks for life changing chaffles!

CPSIA information can be obtained
at www.ICGtesting.com
Printed in the USA
BVHW090332040521
606332BV00006B/1093